Mental health and well-being

By

Kristen B. Medrano

TABLE OF CONTENT

Introduction

In today's fast-paced and interconnected world, it is becoming increasingly evident that mental health holds paramount importance. The way we think, feel, and perceive the world around us shapes our experiences and influences our overall well-being. Mental health is not a mere afterthought; it is the very foundation upon which we build our lives.

A. Opening statement and the importance of mental health:

Imagine a world where every individual thrives emotionally, where compassion and understanding are at the core of our interactions, and where mental well-being is as valued as physical health. Such a world is not just a distant utopia; it is an achievable reality, and it begins with recognizing the importance of mental health. It is essential to acknowledge that mental health affects every aspect of our lives, from our relationships and productivity to our physical health and overall happiness.

B. Definition of mental health and well-being:

What exactly do we mean by mental health and well-being? Mental health encompasses our emotional, psychological, and social well-being. It affects how we think, feel, and act, as well as how we handle stress, relate to others, and make choices. Mental well-being, on the other hand, represents a state of optimal functioning, where individuals can flourish and reach their full potential, even in the face of challenges.

C. Significance of addressing mental health in today's society:

In today's society, the significance of addressing mental health can hardly be overstated. We are witnessing a rising tide of mental health challenges, affecting individuals across age groups, socioeconomic backgrounds, and cultures. Stress, anxiety, depression, and other mental health disorders have become pervasive, leading to profound personal suffering, strained relationships, and diminished productivity. The impact is felt not only by individuals but also by families, communities, and society at large.

D. Purpose and scope of the book:

The purpose of this book is to delve into the multifaceted realm of mental health and well-being, offering a comprehensive understanding of the subject and equipping readers with the knowledge and tools to nurture their own mental well-being. Moreover, it seeks to foster a broader conversation about mental health in today's society and inspire collective action toward creating a more compassionate and inclusive world for everyone.

Throughout the pages of this book, we will explore the various dimensions of mental health, debunk myths and misconceptions, discuss common mental health disorders, delve into strategies for promoting mental well-being, examine the connection between mental and physical health, and delve into the importance of seeking help and overcoming barriers to care. Additionally, we will address the significance of supporting others on their mental health journeys and highlight future directions in the field.

By embarking on this exploration together, we hope to raise awareness, reduce stigma, and empower individuals to prioritize their mental health. The journey toward mental well-being begins here, with the turning of these pages, and it is our sincerest hope that this book will serve as a guiding light, illuminating the path toward a healthier, happier, and more mentally resilient future.

Chapter 1

Understanding Mental Health

A. Overview of Mental Health Disorders

In order to foster a deeper understanding of mental health, it is crucial to gain insight into the wide range of mental health disorders that individuals may face. Mental health disorders encompass a diverse spectrum, each with its own unique set of symptoms, challenges, and treatment approaches.

Within this chapter, we will explore some of the most common mental health disorders, including but not limited to depression, anxiety disorders, bipolar disorder, schizophrenia, eating disorders, substance abuse, and post-traumatic stress disorder (PTSD). By examining these disorders, we can begin to recognize the complexities and nuances of mental health and better comprehend the impact they have on individuals, families, and communities.

B. Causes and Risk Factors

Mental health disorders do not arise in isolation; they are influenced by a combination of causes and risk factors. It is essential to delve into the factors that contribute to the development of mental health disorders to gain a comprehensive understanding of their origins.

Causes of mental health disorders can be multifaceted and may include a combination of genetic, biological, environmental, and psychological factors. Genetic predispositions, imbalances in brain chemistry, traumatic experiences, chronic stress, and social factors such as discrimination or social isolation can all play a role in the onset of mental health disorders. Exploring these causes will shed light on the complexities of mental health and challenge any oversimplified notions.

C. Common Myths and Misconceptions about Mental Health

Unfortunately, mental health is plagued by numerous myths and misconceptions, which contribute to stigma, discrimination, and hinder individuals from seeking help. It is essential to dispel these myths and foster a more accurate and compassionate understanding of mental health.

Some prevalent myths include the notion that mental health disorders are a sign of weakness or personal failure, that individuals with mental health disorders are inherently dangerous, or that seeking treatment is unnecessary. By addressing these misconceptions head-on, we can promote a more inclusive and empathetic society, where mental health is treated with the same importance as physical health.

D. Impact of Mental Health on Individuals, Families, and Communities

Mental health extends beyond individual experiences; it has a profound impact on the well-being of families and communities as well. Understanding the wide-reaching consequences of mental health disorders is crucial for cultivating empathy, support, and appropriate interventions.

At an individual level, mental health disorders can manifest in a variety of ways, affecting emotions, thoughts, behaviors, and overall functioning. Relationships may be strained, work or academic performance may suffer, and individuals may experience a diminished sense of self-worth and fulfillment. Within families, mental health disorders can create stress, disruption, and challenges in maintaining healthy dynamics and communication. On a larger scale, communities may face economic burdens, increased healthcare costs, and reduced productivity due to untreated or unaddressed mental health issues.

By comprehending the far-reaching impact of mental health, we can recognize the urgency of addressing these challenges and work towards creating supportive environments that prioritize mental well-being.

Mental health and well-being

We explored an overview of mental health disorders, delved into the causes and risk factors that contribute to their development, debunked common myths and misconceptions, and examined the impact of mental health on individuals, families, and communities.

By establishing this foundation of knowledge, we can now venture further into the intricacies of mental health and well-being, equipping ourselves with the tools necessary to foster personal growth, promote understanding, and advocate for positive change. As we proceed, we will delve into strategies for promoting mental well-being, seeking help, and building resilient and supportive communities. Together, we can pave the way towards a future where mental health is recognized, valued, and prioritized.

Chapter 2

Promoting Mental Well-being

A. Building Resilience and Coping Skills

Resilience is the ability to adapt, bounce back, and thrive in the face of adversity. Building resilience is a vital component of promoting mental well-being. In this chapter, we will explore strategies and techniques for developing resilience and coping skills.

We will delve into the importance of fostering a positive mindset, cultivating optimism, and reframing challenges as opportunities for growth. Additionally, we will discuss the significance of building a strong support system, seeking professional help when needed, and developing problem-solving and decision-making skills. By equipping ourselves with these tools, we can navigate life's inevitable hardships with greater resilience and emerge stronger on the other side.

B. Practicing Self-care and Stress Management Techniques

Self-care and stress management are fundamental pillars of mental well-being. Taking care of ourselves physically, emotionally, and mentally is essential for maintaining a healthy balance and preventing burnout. This chapter will explore various self-care practices and stress management techniques.

We will delve into the importance of adequate sleep, nutrition, and exercise for overall well-being. We will also discuss relaxation techniques, such as mindfulness, deep breathing exercises, and meditation, which can help alleviate stress and promote mental clarity. Furthermore, we will explore the benefits of engaging in hobbies, practicing creativity, and setting healthy boundaries in our personal and professional lives. By prioritizing self-care and adopting effective stress management techniques, we can nurture our mental well-being and build resilience in the face of daily challenges.

C. Developing Healthy Relationships and Social Support Networks

Human connection and healthy relationships are integral to our mental well-being. In this chapter, we will explore the significance of developing and maintaining healthy relationships and social support networks.

We will discuss effective communication skills, active listening, and empathy, which are essential for fostering meaningful connections. We will also delve into the importance of setting boundaries, resolving conflicts, and seeking support when needed. Additionally, we will examine the benefits of engaging in social activities, volunteering, and participating in community groups to establish a sense of belonging and connection. By nurturing healthy relationships and fostering social support networks, we create a foundation of support and resilience in our lives.

D. Nurturing Emotional Intelligence and Self-Awareness

Emotional intelligence and self-awareness are crucial components of mental well-being. Understanding and managing our emotions effectively, as well as having a deep awareness of ourselves, enables us to navigate life's challenges with greater clarity and emotional resilience.

In this chapter, we will explore the concept of emotional intelligence, which encompasses recognizing and understanding emotions in ourselves and others. We will discuss strategies for managing and regulating emotions, enhancing empathy and interpersonal skills, and developing emotional resilience. Additionally, we will delve into the importance of self-awareness, including recognizing our strengths and limitations, identifying our values and goals, and practicing self-reflection. By nurturing emotional intelligence and self-awareness, we empower ourselves to make healthier choices, build stronger relationships, and cultivate a greater sense of fulfillment and well-being.

Mental health and well-being

By focusing on building resilience and coping skills, practicing self-care and stress management, developing healthy relationships and social support networks, and nurturing emotional intelligence and self-awareness, we can cultivate a strong foundation for our mental well-being.

These practices not only contribute to our individual well-being but also have a ripple effect on our relationships, communities, and society as a whole. As we continue our journey towards mental health and well-being, let us embrace these strategies and incorporate them into our daily lives, allowing them to guide us towards a more balanced and fulfilling existence.

Chapter 3

Mental Health across the Lifespan

A. Mental Health Considerations in Childhood and Adolescence

Childhood and adolescence are critical stages of development, where mental health plays a pivotal role in shaping the trajectory of one's life. In this chapter, we will explore the unique mental health considerations during these formative years.

We will discuss common mental health disorders that may emerge during childhood and adolescence, such as attention-deficit/hyperactivity disorder (ADHD), anxiety disorders, depression, and eating disorders. We will examine the impact of social and academic pressures, family dynamics, and hormonal changes on mental well-being during this stage. Additionally, we will delve into the importance of early intervention, creating supportive environments, and promoting mental health literacy to foster optimal mental well-being in children and adolescents.

B. Mental Health Challenges in Adulthood

Adulthood brings its own set of challenges, and mental health becomes increasingly significant during this stage of life. In this section, we will explore the mental health challenges commonly encountered in adulthood.

We will discuss the impact of work-related stress, financial pressures, relationship dynamics, and societal expectations on mental well-being. We will also examine common mental health disorders experienced during adulthood, such as mood disorders, anxiety disorders, and substance abuse. Additionally, we will explore strategies for managing stress, building resilience, and seeking appropriate support and treatment when needed. By addressing mental health challenges in adulthood, we can foster a more balanced and fulfilling life.

C. Mental Health Issues in the Elderly Population

As individuals age, their mental health needs and challenges may evolve. This section will focus on mental health issues commonly faced by the elderly population.

We will explore the impact of aging, physical health conditions, and life transitions on mental well-being. We will discuss common mental health disorders in the elderly, such as dementia, depression, and loneliness. Additionally, we will examine the importance of social connection, maintaining cognitive stimulation, and providing specialized care and support for the elderly population. By addressing mental health issues in the elderly, we can enhance their quality of life and promote healthy aging.

D. Addressing Mental Health Needs at Each Life Stage

Mental health needs vary at different stages of life, and it is essential to tailor interventions and support accordingly. In this section, we will discuss the importance of addressing mental health needs at each life stage.

We will explore preventive strategies and early intervention in childhood and adolescence to promote mental well-being from an early age. We will also discuss the significance of fostering mental health resilience in adulthood and creating supportive environments that prioritize mental well-being. Moreover, we will delve into the importance of integrating mental health care into elderly care and ensuring accessibility to appropriate support and treatment for the elderly population. By recognizing the unique mental health needs at each life stage, we can develop comprehensive approaches to address mental health challenges effectively.

Mental health and well-being

By understanding and addressing mental health needs across the lifespan, we can promote optimal mental well-being, enhance quality of life, and foster healthy development and aging. As we continue on our journey towards mental health and well-being, let us remain mindful of the unique needs and challenges faced by individuals at different stages of life, providing the support and resources necessary for a mentally healthy and fulfilling existence.

Chapter 4

Common Mental Health Disorders

A. Depression and Anxiety Disorders

Depression and anxiety disorders are among the most prevalent mental health disorders worldwide. In this chapter, we will delve into the nature of these disorders, their symptoms, and available treatment approaches.

We will explore the various types of depression, including major depressive disorder, persistent depressive disorder (dysthymia), and seasonal affective disorder. Additionally, we will discuss anxiety disorders such as generalized anxiety disorder, panic disorder, social anxiety disorder, and specific phobias. By understanding the symptoms, causes, and risk factors associated with these disorders, we can better recognize them in ourselves and others and seek appropriate support and treatment.

B. Bipolar Disorder and Schizophrenia

Bipolar disorder and schizophrenia are complex mental health disorders that significantly impact individuals' lives. In this section, we will explore the characteristics, symptoms, and management of these disorders.

Bipolar disorder is characterized by fluctuations in mood, ranging from manic episodes to depressive episodes. We will discuss the different types of bipolar disorder, the challenges individuals face, and strategies for managing mood swings. Schizophrenia, on the other hand, involves disruptions in perception, thinking, and behavior. We will explore the symptoms, treatment options, and the importance of a comprehensive approach to support individuals with schizophrenia.

C. Eating Disorders and Substance Abuse

Eating disorders and substance abuse are destructive conditions that can severely impact physical and mental health. In this part of the chapter, we will examine these disorders and their implications.

Eating disorders, such as anorexia nervosa, bulimia nervosa, and binge eating disorder, often stem from complex psychological and societal factors. We will discuss the signs, risk factors, and treatment approaches for these disorders, emphasizing the importance of early intervention and multidisciplinary care. Substance abuse, including alcohol and drug addiction, can have devastating effects on individuals' lives. We will explore the causes, consequences, and available treatment options for substance abuse, highlighting the significance of holistic approaches that address underlying mental health issues.

D. Post-Traumatic Stress Disorder (PTSD) and Trauma-Related Conditions

Post-traumatic stress disorder (PTSD) and trauma-related conditions can significantly impact individuals who have experienced traumatic events. In this section, we will delve into these conditions and strategies for healing and recovery.

We will explore the symptoms and diagnostic criteria for PTSD, as well as the psychological and physiological effects of trauma. Furthermore, we will discuss trauma-related conditions, such as acute stress disorder and complex PTSD, which may arise from prolonged or repeated traumatic experiences. We will examine evidence-based treatments and coping strategies for individuals navigating the aftermath of trauma, emphasizing the importance of trauma-informed care and support.

By gaining a deeper understanding of these disorders, their symptoms, and available treatment approaches, we can promote early intervention, reduce stigma, and support individuals on their journey toward mental well-being.

It is important to remember that each individual's experience with these disorders is unique, and treatment approaches should be tailored to their specific needs. By fostering empathy, raising awareness, and providing access to appropriate support and resources, we can create a more inclusive and compassionate society that prioritizes mental health and supports individuals in their recovery and well-being.

Chapter 5

Seeking Help and Treatment

A. Recognizing the Signs and Symptoms of Mental Health Disorders

Recognizing the signs and symptoms of mental health disorders is crucial in seeking help and initiating the path towards treatment. In this chapter, we will explore the common signs and symptoms associated with mental health disorders.

We will discuss the emotional, cognitive, and behavioral indicators that may indicate the presence of a mental health condition. By understanding and recognizing these signs, individuals can better identify when they or their loved ones may be experiencing distress and take proactive steps to seek help and support.

B. Approaches to Diagnosis and Assessment

Accurate diagnosis and assessment are essential in determining the appropriate treatment approach for mental health disorders. In this section, we will delve into the various approaches used in diagnosing and assessing mental health conditions.

We will also discuss the role of mental health professionals, such as psychiatrists, psychologists, and licensed counselors, in conducting assessments and formulating treatment plans based on individual needs. Additionally, we will touch upon the importance of considering cultural, social, and contextual factors when assessing mental health.

C. Overview of Treatment Options (Therapy, Medication, etc.)

This section will provide an overview of the available treatment options for mental health disorders, emphasizing the importance of personalized and holistic approaches.

We will discuss the role of therapy, including various modalities such as cognitive-behavioral therapy (CBT), psychodynamic therapy, and mindfulness-based interventions. We will explore the benefits of therapy in providing a safe and supportive space for individuals to explore their emotions, thoughts, and behaviors. Additionally, we will address the role of medications, when appropriate, in managing certain mental health disorders, highlighting the importance of working closely with a healthcare professional to determine the most suitable treatment plan.

Furthermore, we will touch upon alternative and complementary therapies, self-help strategies, and lifestyle changes that can support overall mental well-being. By understanding the range of treatment options available, individuals can make informed decisions and actively participate in their healing process.

D. Importance of Destigmatizing Mental Health and Seeking Help

Stigma surrounding mental health remains a significant barrier to seeking help and treatment. In this final section, we will emphasize the importance of destigmatizing mental health and encouraging individuals to seek the support they need.

We will explore the negative impact of stigma on individuals, families, and communities, leading to shame, isolation, and reluctance to seek help. We will discuss the role of education, advocacy, and storytelling in challenging misconceptions and promoting empathy and understanding. Moreover, we will highlight the significance of creating supportive environments that foster open conversations about mental health and well-being.

Mental health and well-being

By destigmatizing mental health, we can encourage individuals to seek help without fear of judgment, thus enabling earlier intervention, access to appropriate resources, and improved outcomes. Seeking help is a courageous step towards better mental health, and it is crucial to create a society that embraces and supports those who reach out for assistance.

By increasing awareness, promoting early intervention, and providing access to comprehensive care, we can empower individuals to prioritize their mental well-being and seek the support they need. Let us work collectively to create a society where seeking help for mental health is seen as a sign of strength and where everyone has the opportunity to achieve optimal mental well-being.

Chapter 6

Mental Health and Physical Well-being

A. Connection between Mental and Physical Health

In this chapter, we will explore the intricate relationship between mental and physical health and the impact each has on the other. We will delve into the evidence supporting the connection between mental and physical well-being.

We will discuss how mental health conditions can affect physical health, leading to increased risk of chronic diseases, weakened immune system, and overall reduced quality of life. Likewise, we will examine how physical health problems, such as chronic pain or a serious illness, can impact mental well-being, contributing to symptoms of depression, anxiety, and stress. By recognizing this interconnectedness, we can better understand the importance of addressing both mental and physical health in achieving overall well-being.

B. Impact of Lifestyle Choices on Mental Well-being

The lifestyle choices we make on a daily basis can significantly impact our mental well-being. In this section, we will explore how various lifestyle factors influence our mental health.

We will discuss the importance of regular exercise in promoting mental well-being, as physical activity has been shown to reduce symptoms of anxiety and depression and improve overall mood. Additionally, we will examine the role of nutrition and a balanced diet in supporting brain health and emotional stability. We will also explore the impact of sleep patterns, stress management techniques, and substance use on mental well-being. By making conscious choices that prioritize mental health in our lifestyle, we can enhance our overall well-being.

C. Integrating Mental Health Care into Holistic Healthcare Practices

Holistic healthcare recognizes the importance of addressing mental health alongside physical health. In this part of the chapter, we will explore the integration of mental health care into holistic healthcare practices.

We will discuss the benefits of an integrated approach that considers the whole person, taking into account their mental, physical, emotional, and spiritual well-being. We will explore the importance of collaboration between healthcare providers, including primary care physicians, psychiatrists, psychologists, and other mental health professionals. Additionally, we will examine the value of incorporating mental health screenings and assessments into routine healthcare visits to identify and address mental health concerns early on. By integrating mental health care into holistic healthcare practices, we can promote a comprehensive approach to well-being.

D. Strategies for Promoting a Healthy Mind-Body Balance

Maintaining a healthy mind-body balance is essential for overall well-being. In this section, we will discuss practical strategies and techniques to promote this balance.

We will explore mindfulness and meditation practices that cultivate present-moment awareness, reduce stress, and enhance emotional well-being. We will also discuss relaxation techniques, such as deep breathing exercises and progressive muscle relaxation, that can help individuals manage stress and anxiety. Additionally, we will explore the benefits of engaging in activities that promote joy, creativity, and self-expression, as well as the importance of nurturing social connections and fostering a supportive network. By implementing these strategies, individuals can cultivate a healthy mind-body balance and enhance their overall well-being.

Mental health and well-being

By recognizing the interplay between mental and physical health, making conscious lifestyle choices, integrating mental health into healthcare practices, and adopting strategies that promote balance, individuals can enhance their overall well-being and achieve optimal mental health. Let us prioritize the integration of mental and physical well-being, creating a harmonious and balanced approach to health and leading fulfilling lives.

Chapter 7

Overcoming Barriers to Mental Health Care

A. Socioeconomic and Cultural Factors Affecting Access to Care

Access to mental health care can be hindered by various socioeconomic and cultural factors. In this chapter, we will explore how these factors can create barriers and limit individuals' ability to seek and receive the necessary mental health support.

We will discuss the impact of financial constraints, lack of insurance coverage, and limited healthcare resources on access to mental health care. Additionally, we will explore how cultural beliefs, language barriers, and stigma can further contribute to disparities in accessing mental health services. By understanding these challenges, we can work towards developing strategies to improve access and ensure equitable mental health care for all.

B. Addressing Stigma and Discrimination

Stigma and discrimination surrounding mental health continue to be significant barriers to seeking and receiving mental health care. In this section, we will explore the negative effects of stigma and discrimination and discuss ways to address and challenge them.

We will examine the harmful stereotypes and misconceptions associated with mental health and how they contribute to social stigma. Moreover, we will explore strategies to combat stigma, such as education, public awareness campaigns, and storytelling that humanize the experiences of individuals with mental health conditions. By fostering empathy, understanding, and acceptance, we can create a more inclusive society that supports individuals in seeking the help they need without fear of judgment or discrimination.

C. Promoting Inclusivity and Diversity in Mental Health Services

Inclusive and diverse mental health services are essential to address the unique needs and experiences of individuals from various backgrounds. In this part of the chapter, we will discuss the importance of promoting inclusivity and diversity within mental health care.

We will explore how cultural competence and sensitivity play a crucial role in providing effective mental health support to individuals from diverse communities. We will also discuss the significance of diversifying the mental health workforce, ensuring representation, and addressing the disparities faced by marginalized groups. By creating culturally responsive and inclusive mental health services, we can foster trust, increase accessibility, and improve outcomes for all individuals seeking care.

D. Enhancing Mental Health Literacy in Communities

Mental health literacy empowers individuals to understand, recognize, and respond to mental health challenges effectively. In this section, we will emphasize the importance of enhancing mental health literacy in communities.

We will explore the role of education, awareness campaigns, and community programs in promoting mental health literacy. By providing accurate information about mental health, common disorders, and available resources, we can help individuals make informed decisions about their well-being. Additionally, we will discuss the significance of early intervention and prevention efforts, equipping community members with the knowledge and skills to support their own mental health and that of others.

By addressing these barriers, we can strive towards a more equitable and accessible mental health care system that respects and supports the diverse needs of individuals. Let us work collectively to break down the barriers that prevent individuals from seeking and receiving the mental health care they deserve, fostering a society that values and prioritizes mental well-being for all.

Chapter 8

Supporting Others in Their Mental Health Journeys

A. Strategies for Offering Emotional Support and Empathy

Supporting others in their mental health journeys requires the ability to offer emotional support and empathy. In this chapter, we will explore strategies for providing meaningful support to individuals facing mental health challenges.

We will discuss the importance of active listening, validation, and creating a non-judgmental space for individuals to express their feelings and experiences. We will also explore the power of empathy, understanding, and compassion in helping others feel seen, heard, and supported. By developing these skills, we can foster a sense of connection and provide a valuable source of support for those navigating their mental health journeys.

B. Effective Communication and Active Listening Skills

Effective communication is crucial when supporting others in their mental health journeys. In this section, we will delve into the importance of clear and compassionate communication and active listening.

We will discuss the significance of open-ended questions, reflective listening, and validating emotions to promote a safe and supportive environment for individuals to share their thoughts and feelings. Additionally, we will explore the role of non-verbal communication, such as body language and facial expressions, in conveying empathy and understanding. By honing our communication and active listening skills, we can establish strong foundations for supporting others in their mental health journeys.

C. Providing Resources and Encouraging Help-Seeking Behaviors

Supporting others in their mental health journeys also involves providing them with resources and encouraging help-seeking behaviors. In this part of the chapter, we will discuss strategies for connecting individuals with appropriate resources and fostering a proactive approach to seeking professional help.

We will explore the importance of being knowledgeable about available mental health services, including hotlines, support groups, therapy options, and online resources. We will also discuss the significance of destigmatizing professional help and encouraging individuals to reach out when needed. By providing information and guidance, we can empower others to take the necessary steps towards accessing the support they require.

D. Establishing Boundaries and Self-Care When Supporting Others

Supporting others in their mental health journeys can be emotionally demanding. In this section, we will emphasize the importance of establishing boundaries and practicing self-care to maintain our own well-being while providing support.

We will explore strategies for setting limits, recognizing our own limitations, and practicing self-care activities that help recharge and replenish our emotional reserves. Additionally, we will discuss the importance of seeking our own support systems and resources to ensure we have the necessary support in place while supporting others. By prioritizing our own well-being, we can sustain our ability to provide meaningful support to others over the long term.

By offering emotional support and empathy, developing effective communication and active listening skills, providing resources and encouraging help-seeking behaviors, and establishing boundaries and practicing self-care, we can be a source of strength and support for those navigating their mental health challenges. Let us strive to create a compassionate and supportive community where individuals feel understood, supported, and empowered in their mental health journeys.

Chapter 9

Future Directions in Mental Health

A. Advancements in Mental Health Research and Treatment

The field of mental health is constantly evolving, with ongoing advancements in research and treatment. In this chapter, we will explore the promising developments and future directions in mental health.

We will discuss emerging research findings that deepen our understanding of mental health disorders, their causes, and potential treatment approaches. We will explore innovative therapies, such as neurofeedback, virtual reality, and psychedelic-assisted therapies, that show promise in enhancing mental well-being. Additionally, we will examine the potential of personalized medicine and genetic research in tailoring treatments to individuals' unique needs. By staying abreast of these advancements, we can anticipate a future where mental health care becomes more effective, precise, and accessible.

B. Integrating Technology and Innovation in Mental Health Care

Technology and innovation have the potential to revolutionize mental health care delivery and support. In this section, we will discuss how technology can be integrated into mental health care and its potential benefits.

We will explore the use of telehealth, mobile apps, and online platforms for remote therapy, support groups, and self-help resources. We will also discuss the integration of artificial intelligence and machine learning in mental health assessment, early intervention, and personalized treatment planning. Additionally, we will explore the role of wearable devices and digital biomarkers in monitoring mental well-being and predicting episodes of distress. By embracing technology and innovation, we can expand access to mental health care, enhance self-management tools, and improve outcomes for individuals.

C. Advocacy and Policy Efforts for Mental Health Reform

Advocacy and policy efforts play a vital role in shaping the future of mental health care. In this part of the chapter, we will discuss the importance of advocacy and policy reform to improve mental health services and reduce disparities.

We will explore the need for increased funding and resources for mental health care, as well as the importance of parity laws to ensure equitable coverage for mental health conditions. We will also discuss the significance of DE stigmatization campaigns, public awareness initiatives, and education programs to promote understanding and empathy. By advocating for mental health reform, we can create a society that values and prioritizes mental well-being, leading to improved access to care and better outcomes for all.

D. Encouraging a Compassionate and Inclusive Approach to Mental Health

As we envision the future of mental health, it is essential to foster a compassionate and inclusive approach. In this section, we will discuss the significance of creating a supportive environment that embraces diversity and promotes mental well-being for all.

We will explore the need for culturally responsive and trauma-informed care that recognizes and respects individuals' unique backgrounds and experiences. We will discuss the importance of reducing stigma, discrimination, and societal barriers that hinder individuals from seeking help. Additionally, we will emphasize the value of community support networks, peer support programs, and community-based initiatives in fostering resilience and well-being. By encouraging a compassionate and inclusive approach, we can create a future where everyone feels valued, supported, and empowered in their mental health journeys.

As we look to the future, let us remain optimistic about the possibilities and committed to promoting mental well-being for all. By embracing advancements, advocating for change, and fostering inclusivity, we can shape a future where mental health is prioritized, stigma is eradicated, and access to quality care is a reality for everyone.

Conclusion:

In this book, we have embarked on a comprehensive exploration of mental health and well-being, delving into various aspects that shape our understanding and experiences. Let us take a moment to recap the key points discussed, reiterating their significance in our collective pursuit of mental well-being.

We began by recognizing the importance of mental health, understanding that it is an integral part of our overall well-being. We defined mental health and well-being, acknowledging that they encompass more than just the absence of mental illness. Throughout the book, we emphasized the significance of addressing mental health in today's society, considering the profound impact it has on individuals, families, and communities.

We recognized the diverse range of mental health disorders, exploring their causes, risk factors, and dispelling common myths and misconceptions that hinder understanding and support. We explored the impact of mental health on different stages of life, recognizing the unique challenges and considerations faced by children, adolescents, adults, and the elderly.

We delved into common mental health disorders, understanding the complexities of conditions such as depression, anxiety, bipolar disorder, schizophrenia, eating disorders, substance abuse, and trauma-related conditions. We emphasized the importance of seeking help and treatment, recognizing the signs and symptoms, and promoting mental health literacy in communities.

Moreover, we recognized the intricate connection between mental and physical well-being, exploring lifestyle choices, resilience-building, self-care, and the integration of mental health into holistic healthcare practices. We acknowledged the barriers to mental health care, such as socioeconomic factors, stigma, and discrimination, while emphasizing the need for inclusivity, diversity, and enhanced access to mental health services.

Looking towards the future, we discussed the exciting advancements in mental health research and treatment, the integration of technology and innovation, advocacy and policy efforts for reform, and the significance of fostering a compassionate and inclusive approach. It is our hope that mental health will be treated with the same importance as physical health, with increased understanding, acceptance, and support for individuals on their mental health journeys.

In conclusion, we issue a resounding call to action. Let us prioritize mental health and well-being, recognizing that it is not a journey to embark upon alone. We encourage individuals, families, communities, and policymakers to commit themselves to creating a world that values and supports mental well-being for all. By destigmatizing mental health, promoting awareness, investing in research and treatment, and fostering empathy and understanding, we can reshape the narrative around mental health.

As we close this book, we offer our final thoughts and words of encouragement to all readers. Embrace your mental health journey with courage, compassion, and resilience. Seek support, whether from professionals, loved ones, or support networks. Remember that you are not alone, and there is strength in vulnerability. Prioritize self-care, establish boundaries, and nourish your mind, body, and soul.

May this book serve as a guide, a source of knowledge, and a catalyst for change. Let us collectively create a world where mental health is given the attention, care, and support it deserves. May you embark on your mental health journey with a renewed sense of purpose, hope, and determination. Your well-being matters. Your mental health matters.

Mental health and well-being